A Comprehensive Guide For Stroke Recovery Caregiving

Empowering Caregivers, Nurturing Survivors, A Holistic Approach to Stroke Recovery and Prevention

Maggie E. McDonald

Table of Content

Introduction

Strokes, which are also sometimes referred to as cerebrovascular accidents, is a type of medical emergency that takes place when there is a disturbance in the blood distribution to the brain. This disruption has the potential to result in severe effects, which can range from transitory deficits to impaired skills that are permanent. Understanding the seriousness of strokes and acquiring the skills necessary to offer appropriate treatment is of the utmost importance, not only for those who work in the medical field but also for anyone who could find themselves in a position to provide care for someone else. The purpose of this book is to shed light on the complex phenomena that are strokes, with a particular focus on the necessity of comprehensive care and the provision of a road map for those who are providing care as well as those who are on the road to recovery.

A Brief Explanation of Strokes

The occurrence of a stroke is characterized by a disruption in the blood flow to the brain, which can be caused by either an obstruction in the blood vessels (known as an ischemic stroke) or the rupture of a blood vessel (known as a hemorrhagic stroke). When the brain is deprived of the oxygen and nutrients it needs to function properly, it begins to experience damage that cannot be reversed within minutes. This injury can show in numerous ways, altering speech, mobility, cognition, and other important activities. The two primary forms of strokes, ischemic and hemorrhagic, have unique features but have the potential for disastrous outcomes.

Ischemic strokes, which account for the majority of instances, often arise from the obstruction of blood arteries by clots, debris, or fatty deposits. On the other side, hemorrhagic strokes occur when blood arteries break, producing bleeding within the brain. Both forms necessitate rapid medical intervention to limit additional harm and enhance the chances of recovery.

Importance of Understanding and Providing Care

The relevance of comprehending strokes extends beyond the immediate affected individual to their whole support system. Family members, friends, and caregivers play a significant role in the recovery and well-being of stroke survivors. Knowledge regarding the nature of strokes, their symptoms, and the urgency of obtaining medical treatment is crucial for a fast reaction that can dramatically improve outcomes.

Providing care for someone who has experienced a stroke involves not just medical skills but also empathy, patience, and adaptability. Strokes typically bring up a variety of issues, from physical limitations to emotional and cognitive struggles. Caregivers need to appreciate the varied nature of these difficulties to offer comprehensive care.

Beyond the immediate post-stroke phase, knowing the long-term impact and potential problems is as critical. Effective treatment entails not just treating the immediate aftermath of a stroke but also adapting tactics to the developing requirements of the survivor throughout their recovery journey.

Purpose of the Guide

The purpose of this guide is to serve as a comprehensive resource for caregivers, family members, and anyone involved in the care of stroke survivors. It seeks to bridge the gap between medical knowledge and practical caregiving, offering insights, strategies, and actionable advice.

In the middle of a medical crisis, individuals may feel overwhelmed and unprepared. This book attempts to be a beacon of clarity, providing not just information about strokes and their complications but also assistance on how to handle the problems that come with caring. By demystifying the complexity surrounding strokes and their aftermath, this book encourages caregivers to play a proactive and educated part in the healing process.

Additionally, the handbook is meant to be accessible to a large readership.

Whether you are a healthcare professional trying to expand your understanding of stroke care or a family member thrown into the position of a caregiver, the material offered here is geared to satisfy varied requirements. The ultimate objective is to establish a resource that not only informs but also inspires trust in those responsible for the well-being of stroke survivors.

Understanding Strokes

Unraveling the Complex Tapestry

Strokes, frequently seen as a silent and abrupt aggressor, is a substantial public health problem globally. Delving into the complicated arena of strokes includes identifying their kinds, appreciating their causes, and acknowledging the vast array of risk factors that contribute to their occurrence. This section acts as a compass, navigating through the definitions, kinds, causes, and contextual factors concerning strokes.

Definition and Types of Strokes

At its root, a stroke is a disturbance in the blood flow to the brain, leading to a cascade of events that can result in irreparable damage to brain tissue. Understanding the kinds of strokes is crucial for creating appropriate responses and treatment techniques.

1. Ischemic Strokes:

Ischemic strokes account for roughly 80% of all stroke cases. They unfold when the blood veins supplying the brain get clogged, preventing the passage of oxygen and critical nutrients. The blockage frequently comes from blood clots, fatty deposits, or debris that hinder the veins, ending in deprivation of circulation to certain brain areas. This deprivation produces a cascade effect, commencing the degeneration of brain cells within minutes.

2. Hemorrhagic Strokes:

Hemorrhagic strokes, however less prevalent, are defined by bleeding within the brain. This bleeding originates from the rupture of blood vessels, producing greater pressure and potentially inflicting extensive harm. Factors such as uncontrolled high blood pressure, aneurysms, or trauma might contribute to the incidence of hemorrhagic strokes. The urgent urgency of these strokes is highlighted by the necessity to reduce the pressure on the brain rapidly.

Causes and Risk Factors

Understanding the fundamental causes and risk factors connected with strokes uncovers the complexity of this medical issue. Strokes are typically not discrete occurrences but rather a confluence of several variables that merge to form a perfect storm. Unraveling these aspects is vital for preventive treatment.

1. Lifestyle Related Factors:

Lifestyle decisions have a tremendous effect on stroke risk. Factors such as obesity, physical inactivity, and excessive alcohol use lead to the development of illnesses including hypertension, diabetes, and high cholesterol   all of which are important precursors to strokes. Smoking, with its adverse influence on blood arteries, is another modifiable risk factor that deserves consideration in stroke prevention methods.

2. Medical Conditions:

Several medical problems heighten the risk of strokes. High blood pressure, sometimes termed the "silent killer," stands as a key cause. Conditions like atrial fibrillation, a heart rhythm condition, can lead to the production of blood clots that may travel to the brain, producing a stroke. Diabetes, defined by increased blood sugar levels, substantially increases the risk by weakening blood vessels over time.

3. Age, Race, and Gender Considerations:

Age is an unquestionable component in stroke risk, with persons over 55 experiencing a heightened sensitivity.

Furthermore, racial and gender issues contribute to the stroke landscape. African American and Hispanic persons are likely to face a larger risk than their peers of other racial or ethnic origins. Men, overall, have a larger risk of strokes than women, however, women have additional hazards related to hormonal variables, particularly throughout certain life phases.

4. The Role of COVID-19:

In the ever-evolving spectrum of health problems, the function of COVID-19 in stroke risk has arisen as a focus of research. Early study reveals a potential relationship between COVID-19 infection and an elevated risk of ischemic strokes. The virus's influence on the vascular system and its tendency for blood clot formation may contribute to this heightened risk. However, further study is necessary to completely grasp the subtleties of this interaction.

Understanding these complex causes and risk factors is like unraveling the numerous threads of a tapestry. Each aspect, linked together, gives a thorough picture of the variables contributing to strokes. Armed with this information, individuals and healthcare professionals alike may engage on the road of prevention and early intervention, seeking to disentangle the complexity that surrounds strokes.

Recognizing Stroke Symptoms

In the area of stroke care, time is not simply of the essence; it's the linchpin that may decide the course of recovery. Recognizing the signs of a stroke immediately is analogous to holding the key to a door beyond which lies the prospect for timely intervention and reduced harm. This section acts as a lighthouse, casting light on the different signs that indicate a stroke and underlining the crucial significance of rapid intervention.

Overview of Common Symptoms

Strokes, frequently referred to as "brain attacks," reveal their existence with a constellation of symptoms that necessitate quick attention. Recognizing these signs is the first critical step toward preventing the potentially disastrous effects of a stroke.

1. FAST Acronym:

The FAST acronym is a mnemonic scheme that encompasses the major indicators of a stroke, acting as a rapid and remembered reference for both healthcare professionals and the general public.

Face Drooping:

One of the defining indicators of a stroke is asymmetry in facial features. A person undergoing a stroke may demonstrate drooping on one side of their face, making it seem uneven when they attempt to smile.

Arm Weakness:

Stroke-induced weakness commonly appears in one arm. Asking the person to extend both arms and monitoring whether one arm slips lower might give a significant hint.

Speech Difficulties:

Impairments in speech or unexpected difficulties in expressing words are typical in stroke scenarios. Slurred speech or the inability to grasp or answer clearly may be suggestive of a stroke.

Time to Call for Help:

Time is the linchpin. If any of the aforementioned indicators are seen, it is vital to seek emergency medical care without delay. Every passing minute without action raises the chance of permanent harm.

2. Other Symptoms:

While the FAST acronym simply encapsulates major signs, strokes can present in several ways, each needing attention and rapid intervention.

Headache:

A sudden, terrible headache, sometimes characterized as the "worst headache of one's life," can be an indication of a stroke. The quick development of significant head discomfort should not be discounted and needs prompt medical treatment.

Trouble Walking:

Coordination and balance are commonly affected by a stroke. Individuals may feel abrupt dizziness, loss of balance, or trouble walking. Observing any inexplicable decrease in movement is vital for diagnosing a potential stroke.

These symptoms combined create a clear image of the urgency that surrounds stroke situations. Beyond the physical symptoms, strokes can also impair cognitive functioning, confusing, abrupt visual changes, and trouble in interpreting or processing information.

Importance of Timely Intervention

The criticality of quick action in the face of a suspected stroke cannot be stressed. The significance of time on treatment success is a guiding principle in stroke care, embodied in the slogan "Time is Brain." This theory underlines the reality that with every passing minute without adequate medical intervention, brain cells are in danger of irreparable damage.

1. The Golden Window:

The initial few hours, frequently referred to as the "golden window," are critical in stroke therapy. During this phase, particular actions, such as delivering clot-busting drugs or performing surgeries to remove clots, can be most beneficial.

Beyond this time, the potential for reaching ideal outcomes declines.

2. Clot Busting Medications:

For ischemic strokes, which originate from blood clots, providing drugs such as tissue plasminogen activator (tPA) can help break clots and restore blood flow to the brain. However, the administration of these drugs is time-sensitive, stressing the necessity for prompt identification and management.

3. Endovascular Procedures:

In certain circumstances, endovascular techniques, such as thrombectomy, may be performed to physically remove clots from the blood arteries. Again, the success of these procedures rests on quick response.

4. Reducing Long-Term Disability:

Timely intervention not only raises the chances of survival but also dramatically minimizes the likelihood of long-term impairment. Stroke survivors who get quick and proper care are more likely to regain functioning and report a smoother recovery trajectory.

In essence, time becomes a costly commodity when strokes are in play. Recognizing the symptoms swiftly and obtaining emergency medical care without delay is not only a question of urgency; it is a critical component that can influence the path of a person's life in the aftermath of a stroke.

As we navigate through the intricacies of stroke treatment, the detection of signs and the requirement of immediate action stands as sentinel principles. The ensuing parts will unravel the diagnostic processes, medicinal therapies, and post-stroke care strategies, providing a full tapestry of information to help both caregivers and healthcare professionals in the world of stroke recovery and prevention.

Medical Emergency and Initial Response

In the face of a stroke, every passing second bears tremendous ramifications for the individual's well-being. The quickness and accuracy of the initial response become the fulcrum that can determine the trajectory of recovery. This section serves as a guide, highlighting the crucial phases in the medical emergency and the early aftermath of a stroke.

Calling for Emergency Medical Assistance

1. Immediate Action Saves Lives:

The beginning of emergency medical help is not only a smart measure; it is a life-saving requirement. Dialing medical assistance promptly upon identifying the signs of a stroke sets in motion a series of actions that can be crucial in limiting the impact of the stroke.

2. Provide Clear Information:

When calling medical assistance, clarity is crucial. Providing precise and concise information regarding the observed symptoms, the individual's present state, and any relevant medical history can enable emergency responders to arrange the required resources and actions.

3. Stay on the Line:

Emergency dispatchers may ask questions to determine the severity of the issue and give direction. It is crucial to stay on the line, follow their directions, and not hang up until asked to do so. This enables a constant channel of contact for real-time information and help.

4. Share the FAST Assessment:

If the FAST assessment has been done and identifies indicators of a stroke (Face drooping, Arm weakness, Speech difficulty, Time to call for help), sending this information to the emergency dispatcher helps speed the response procedure. Time is of the essence and every second matters.

Providing Comfort and Reassurance

1. Maintain Calmness:

In the middle of a medical emergency, maintaining calm is a vital element of offering good help. A calm and controlled manner might not only reassure the individual suffering the stroke but also promote clearer communication with healthcare providers.

2. Ensure Safety:

Prioritize safety in the local environment. Remove any possible risks or obstructions that can represent a risk to the individual or those offering help. Creating a safe area is important for both immediate treatment and the following arrival of emergency medical services.

3. Offer Emotional Support:

A stroke may be a terrifying and bewildering event for the individual afflicted. Offering words of comfort and encouragement might help ease anxiety. Simple remarks conveying encouragement and the confidence that aid is on the way may make a tremendous impact in the individual's state of mind.

4. Do Not Delay for Self Transport:

It is vital not to try self-transport to the hospital. Emergency medical services are prepared with the necessary equipment and staff to give rapid care on route to the hospital. Waiting for their arrival guarantees that the individual receives proper and timely medical treatment.

Notifying Healthcare Professionals About Symptoms and Recent Medical History

1. Share Critical Information:

Upon the arrival of emergency medical professionals, rapidly disclose any pertinent information regarding the observed symptoms and the individual's recent medical history. This can include pre-existing illnesses, medicines, and any recent occurrences that would be significant to the case.

2. Facilitate Communication:

Be prepared to answer inquiries from healthcare providers on the beginning of symptoms, any known medical issues, and the individual's response to the initial symptoms. Clear and succinct communication assists in the rapid and correct appraisal of the issue.

3. Provide Medication Information:

If the client is taking any drugs, offer specifics to the healthcare providers. This information is vital for ensuring that suitable medical interventions and therapies correspond with the individual's existing medical regimen.

4. Advocate for the Patient:

In the earliest stages of a medical emergency, the individual afflicted may be bewildered or unable to communicate their medical history. Serving as an advocate by giving critical information helps bridge this gap, permitting a more efficient and educated response.

As the first reaction unfolds, the joint efforts of emergency medical services, caregivers, and healthcare professionals set the foundation for following treatments. Recognizing the urgency of a stroke, promptly activating emergency services, and offering immediate comfort constitute a coherent triangle that attempts to optimize the odds of a happy result.

Diagnosis and Treatment

Navigating the Path to Recovery

In the convoluted environment of stroke treatment, rapid and precise diagnosis lays the groundwork for individualized therapies that can alter the trajectory of recovery. This section acts as a compass, directing us through the diagnostic methods performed in the aftermath of a stroke and the diversity of medical measures that form the cornerstone of effective therapy.

Overview of Diagnostic Procedures

1. CT Scans, MRI, and Other Imaging Tests:

CT Scans (Computed Tomography):

CT scans are generally the initial diagnostic technique used to check a person suspected of having a stroke. These scans give precise images of the brain, enabling healthcare experts to identify regions affected by the stroke and evaluate whether it is ischemic or hemorrhagic. The speed and accessibility of CT scans make them helpful in the time-sensitive situation of stroke diagnosis.

MRI (Magnetic Resonance Imaging):

MRI is another strong imaging tool that delivers precise views of the brain's anatomy. While not typically the first option in the acute phase of a stroke, MRI can give important insights, notably in discriminating between old and fresh strokes. It is particularly important in determining the level of damage and directing long-term therapy plans.

Angiography and Other Imaging Modalities:

Angiography, combining the use of contrast dye and imaging methods, can reveal blood arteries in the brain. This helps identify any anomalies, such as blood clots or vascular malformations, leading to the stroke. Other imaging modalities, such as Doppler ultrasonography, may be applied to monitor blood flow and locate possible obstructions.

2. Blood Tests:

Complete Blood Count (CBC):

Blood tests, particularly a complete blood count (CBC), assist in identifying several variables that could contribute to stroke risk. Anemia, infection, and some blood diseases can be discovered by blood analysis, affording vital information into the general health state of the individual.

Coagulation Studies:

Coagulation tests, such as the prothrombin time (PT) and activated partial thromboplastin time (aPTT), measure the blood's clotting capabilities. Abnormalities in coagulation might signal to disorders that may require specialized therapies, notably in the context of ischemic strokes.

Lipid Profile:

Measuring lipid levels, especially cholesterol, is critical in understanding cardiovascular health. Elevated cholesterol levels can lead to atherosclerosis, a significant cause of ischemic strokes. Managing lipid levels by lifestyle modifications or drugs is a crucial element of stroke prevention.

Medical Interventions and Medications

1. Clot Busting Drugs:

Tissue Plasminogen Activator (tPA):

In the area of ischemic strokes, when a clot obstructs blood flow to the brain, clot-busting medications like tissue plasminogen activator (tPA) play a vital role. Administered intravenously, tPA acts by dissolving the clot, restoring blood flow, and perhaps reducing damage to the brain. Time is a significant aspect in the usage of tPA, with a precise window of efficacy within the first few hours following symptom start.

Endovascular Thrombectomy:

In rare circumstances, especially when the clot is in a big artery, endovascular thrombectomy may be done. This treatment includes the insertion of a catheter into the blood arteries to physically remove the clot. Endovascular treatments are typically recommended when clot-busting drugs alone may not be adequate.

2. Antiplatelet and Anticoagulant Medications:

Aspirin:

Aspirin, an antiplatelet medicine, is routinely recommended to persons who have undergone an ischemic stroke or a transient ischemic attack (TIA). By suppressing platelet aggregation and lowering the production of blood clots, aspirin acts as a preventative strategy against recurrent strokes.

Clopidogrel (Plavix):

Clopidogrel, another antiplatelet medicine, may be given in conjunction with or as an alternative to aspirin, depending on individual circumstances. It works by preventing platelets from adhering together and creating clots.

Warfarin and Direct Oral Anticoagulants (DOACs):

For patients with certain disorders, such as atrial fibrillation, which raises the risk of clot formation in the heart, anticoagulant drugs like warfarin or DOACs may be administered. These drugs interfere with the blood clotting process, lowering the probability of stroke.

Dabigatran, Rivaroxaban, Apixaban, Edoxaban:

Direct Oral Anticoagulants (DOACs) constitute a novel family of anticoagulant drugs that provide benefits over older agents like warfarin. They normally do not require frequent monitoring and are associated with a decreased risk of bleeding problems.

Each diagnostic method and medicinal intervention serves a particular function in the full landscape of stroke treatment. From the fast clarity afforded by imaging tests to the focused impact of clot-busting therapies and anticoagulant medications, these treatments are planned to limit damage, boost recovery, and avoid future strokes.

Post-Stroke Care

Nurturing Recovery, and Embracing Resilience

The process of stroke recovery stretches long beyond the early moments of diagnosis and therapy. Post-stroke treatment provides a critical chapter in this tale, distinguished by hospitalization, rehabilitation, medication management, and the sensitive handling of emotional and psychological components. It is a continuum where each phase contributes to the individual's resilience and the goal of optimal recovery.

Hospitalization and Initial Recovery

1. Specialized Stroke Units:

Hospitalization following a stroke is not only a necessity; it is a purposeful decision aimed at providing expert treatment. Many hospitals have specific stroke units equipped with experts experienced in stroke care. This concentrated approach guarantees that people receive individualized interventions, monitoring, and support.

2. Monitoring and Assessments:

During the first healing period, constant monitoring is necessary. Regular assessments, particularly neurological exams, assist in quantifying the level of damage, track improvement, and drive the formulation of tailored treatment plans. Monitoring vital signs, addressing potential difficulties, and taking preventative actions are key components of this period.

3. Multidisciplinary Team Approach:

The intricacy of stroke rehabilitation necessitates a multidisciplinary team approach. Neurologists, nurses, physical therapists, occupational therapists, speech therapists, and psychologists work to treat multiple elements of the individual's well being. This thorough method maximizes the odds of a smoother recovery trajectory.

Rehabilitation and Therapy Options

1. Physical Therapy:

Restoring Mobility and Functionality:

Physical therapy plays a major part in post-stroke recovery. Tailored exercise regimens attempt to restore mobility, enhance strength, and address difficulties such as balance and coordination. Individuals engage with physical therapists to restore control over afflicted limbs and boost overall physical function.

Gait Training:

For people experiencing trouble walking or keeping balance, gait training becomes a key topic. This incorporates focused workouts and activities aimed at improving walking patterns and minimizing the risk of falls.

Assistive Devices:

Physical therapists may introduce assistance equipment such as canes or walkers to help mobility throughout the healing process. These tools give help and promote freedom while navigating daily routines.

2. Occupational Therapy:

Daily Living Skills:

Occupational therapy focuses on strengthening an individual's capacity to conduct daily activities. This includes duties such as clothing, grooming, cooking, and other basic activities of daily living (ADLs).

Therapists interact with individuals to design solutions that accommodate any physical or cognitive obstacles.

Adaptive Techniques:

Occupational therapists provide adaptive approaches and instruments that ease activities. From adapted utensils to customized equipment, these treatments permit individuals to engage in meaningful activities with improved freedom.

3. Speech Therapy:

Communication Skills:

Speech therapy tackles issues associated with speech and swallowing. For people suffering from difficulty in speech or language understanding, therapists offer activities to develop communication abilities. Additionally, therapies focus on strengthening swallowing function to lower the risk of aspiration.

Cognitive Rehabilitation:

Cognitive components, including memory, concentration, and problem solving, are also addressed in speech therapy. Cognitive rehabilitation activities attempt to boost cognitive function and help patients in recovering mental sharpness.

Medication Management and Adherence

1. Optimizing Medication Regimens:

Post stroke treatment generally entails continuing drug management. Individuals may be offered drugs to address risk factors such as hypertension, diabetes, or increased cholesterol levels. Adherence to prescribed drugs is crucial for long term stroke prevention and general health.

2. Anticoagulant and Antiplatelet Therapy:

Those at risk of recurrent strokes, especially adults with atrial fibrillation, may be administered anticoagulant medicines. These medications, such as warfarin or direct oral anticoagulants (DOACs), inhibit the development of blood clots. Anti-platelet drugs like aspirin or clopidogrel may also be part of the post-stroke therapeutic regimen.

3. Regular Monitoring and Adjustments:

Regular follow-up consultations with healthcare specialists are needed to check the efficacy and safety of prescription drugs. Adjustments to pharmaceutical regimens may be changed based on the individual's reaction and any changes in health state.

Addressing Emotional and Psychological Aspects

1. Emotional Impact of Stroke:

The aftermath of a stroke generally accompanies a flood of emotions, ranging from annoyance and worry to loss and melancholy. Acknowledging and resolving these emotional complexities is an important element of post-stroke treatment. Healthcare experts, including psychologists and counselors, may be involved to give support and assistance.

2. Counseling and Support Groups:

Engaging in individual or group therapy sessions can give a secure environment for individuals to express their concerns and negotiate the emotional consequences of stroke. Support groups, containing persons with similar experiences, create a sense of connection and shared understanding.

3. Depression and Anxiety Management:

Post stroke melancholy and anxiety are not uncommon. Healthcare providers may offer therapy methods or, in certain situations, drugs to manage these mental well-being. Recognizing and managing emotional well being is crucial to creating a comprehensive recovery.

4. Family and Caregiver Support:

The emotional burden of stroke extends to family members and caregivers. Providing tools and support for caregivers, including respite care alternatives and educational programs, helps the overall well-being of both the individual recovering from the stroke and those supporting them.

In the tapestry of post-stroke care, each thread reflects a distinct dimension of rehabilitation. From the physical healing supported by rehabilitation to the rigorous control of pharmaceuticals and the subtle addressing of emotional well-being, this continuum epitomizes resilience, adaptation, and the collaborative quest of a life characterized by strength and hope.

Lifestyle Modifications for Stroke Prevention

Empowering Health and Wellness

Stroke prevention is not only a duty for the domain of drugs; it is a comprehensive undertaking woven into the fabric of daily living. This section goes into lifestyle adjustments that act as pillars in the prevention of strokes. From nutritional advice to the encouragement of physical exercise, controlling risk factors, and embracing healthy behaviors, each component plays a key part in empowering individuals on the road of stroke prevention.

Dietary Recommendations

1. Embracing a Heart Healthy Diet:

The cornerstone of stroke prevention is formed in the decisions we make at the dinner table. A heart-healthy diet, rich in fruits, vegetables, whole grains, and lean meats, adds to overall cardiovascular well-being. Prioritizing nutrient-dense foods above processed ones forms the cornerstone of dietary recommendations.

2. Reducing Sodium Intake:

Excessive salt consumption is connected to hypertension, a major risk factor for strokes. By actively lowering salt intake, individuals can better regulate blood pressure levels. Choosing fresh, whole foods over processed ones and adding herbs and spices for flavor boost the nutritional content of meals while minimizing salt consumption.

3. Moderating Saturated and Trans Fats:

Saturated and trans fats lead to the buildup of cholesterol in the arteries, increasing the risk of atherosclerosis and, subsequently, strokes. Choosing healthy fats, such as those found in avocados, almonds, and olive oil, and reducing the intake of saturated and trans fats found in fried meals and processed snacks coincides with stroke prevention aims.

4. Incorporating Omega 3 Fatty Acids:

Omega 3 fatty acids, present in fatty fish like salmon and mackerel, walnuts, and flaxseeds, have been connected with cardiovascular benefits. Including these sources of omega 3s in the diet may contribute to the lowering of stroke risk by supporting heart health.

Exercise and Physical Activity

1. Aerobic Exercise for Cardiovascular Health:

Regular physical activity is an effective ally in the prevention of strokes. Aerobic workouts, such as brisk walking, running, swimming, or cycling, help to cardiovascular health by boosting blood circulation, decreasing blood pressure, and promoting general fitness.

2. Strength Training for Muscle Health:

In addition to aerobic activity, adding strength training exercises helps preserve muscle mass and contributes to overall physical well being. Strong muscles maintain joint health and contribute to functional fitness, minimizing the incidence of falls and related injuries.

3. Flexibility and Balance Exercises:

Activities that enhance flexibility and balance are vital components of a well-rounded fitness regimen. Yoga and tai chi, for example, not only develop physical flexibility but also boost emotional well-being. Improved balance minimizes the chance of falls, an important concern in stroke prevention.

4. Consistency and Enjoyment:

The key to keeping an active lifestyle resides on consistency and enjoyment. Finding activities that offer delight and can be smoothly integrated into daily life boosts the chance of commitment. Whether it's dancing, gardening, or engaging in group sports, the objective is to make physical exercise a sustainable and meaningful part of life.

Managing Blood Pressure and Other Risk Factors

1. Regular Blood Pressure Monitoring:

Hypertension is a prominent risk factor for strokes. Regular monitoring of blood pressure levels and, if necessary, medication adherence as suggested by healthcare professionals are key components of stroke prevention. Lifestyle alterations, including dietary changes and exercise, have a crucial role in regulating blood pressure.

2. Diabetes Management:

Individuals with diabetes suffer an increased risk of strokes. Effective control of diabetes by medication, lifestyle adjustments, and regular monitoring of blood sugar levels is critical in stroke prevention. Maintaining a healthy weight and adopting a balanced diet contribute to diabetes control.

3. Cholesterol Control:

Elevated cholesterol levels contribute to atherosclerosis, a condition where arteries get constricted and may lead to strokes. Lifestyle alterations, including dietary changes and the use of cholesterol lowering drugs if indicated, contribute to cholesterol management. Regular checkups and lipid profile evaluations guide treatments.

4. Weight Management:

Maintaining a healthy weight is not just about beauty; it is a vital part of stroke prevention. Obesity is connected to several risk factors, including hypertension, diabetes, and cardiovascular disease. Combining a good diet with frequent physical activity improves weight control and general health.

Smoking Cessation and Alcohol Moderation

1. Quitting Smoking:

Smoking is a powerful risk factor for strokes. The chemicals in tobacco smoke lead to the constriction of blood arteries, increased blood clotting, and the development of atherosclerosis. Quitting smoking is a critical step in stroke prevention. Support systems, including counseling and nicotine replacement medications, can assist in the quitting process.

2. Moderating Alcohol Consumption:

While moderate alcohol use has been associated with certain cardiovascular advantages, excessive alcohol intake has health hazards, including an increased risk of strokes. Moderation is crucial, with guidelines advising that, if persons want to use alcohol, it should be done in moderation. For most adults, this amounts to up to one drink per day for women and up to two drinks per day for men.

Holistic Empowerment for Stroke Prevention

In the complicated ballet of lifestyle adjustments, each step is a proclamation of agency and empowerment. From the attentive decisions made at the dinner table to the rhythmic cadence of regular physical exercise, these lifestyle adjustments function as instruments in the symphony of stroke prevention. By accepting these concepts, individuals not only minimize their risk of strokes but also develop a foundation for enduring health and well-being. The road towards a stroke-free future is a dynamic collaboration between educated decisions and the tenacity of the human spirit.

Home Care for Stroke Survivors

The shift from hospital to home after a stroke represents a key milestone in the process of rehabilitation. Home care becomes a vital factor in assisting stroke patients as they regain their independence and handle the obstacles of everyday living. In this section, we discuss the key features of home care, comprising the alteration of the living environment for safety, aid with everyday tasks, medication administration, and watchful monitoring for indicators of difficulties.

Modifying the Living Environment for Safety

1. Adapting to New Realities:

The house is a refuge, and its modification becomes crucial in guaranteeing the safety and comfort of stroke survivors. Simple adjustments may have a huge effect. Installing handrails in crucial locations, such as corridors and toilets, gives vital support for movement. The elimination of tripping risks and maintaining enough illumination are smart actions that contribute to a safer living environment.

2. Accessible Living Spaces:

Creating living areas that are accessible and adaptable is key to encouraging independence. Doorways should be wide enough to accept mobility assistance, and furniture placement should allow for simple navigation. Installing ramps or lifts, if needed, ensures that every section of the home is within reach. These adjustments permit stroke patients to walk freely within their familiar settings.

3. Assistive Devices and Technologies:

The integration of assistive gadgets and smart technology further enriches the home environment. From the installation of grab bars in the bathroom to the inclusion of smart home gadgets that allow remote control of lighting and appliances, these items contribute not only to safety but also to convenience. Empowering stroke survivors with these tools creates a sense of autonomy.

Assisting with Daily Activities

1. Personal Care Assistance:

The process of rehabilitation sometimes entails the need for support with personal care duties. Caregivers play a significant role in giving help for routines such as washing, dressing, and grooming. This aid is not only practical but also a chance to protect the individual's dignity and sense of self.

2. Mobility Support:

Depending on the amount of movement issues, stroke survivors may utilize mobility aids such as canes, walkers, or wheelchairs. Caregivers help by supplying assistance when needed, ensuring the precise adjustment of mobility aids for stability, and encouraging safe movement. This assistance helps stroke patients to manage their home area with confidence.

3. Meal Preparation and Nutrition:

Nutrition is a cornerstone of rehabilitation. Caregivers play a critical role in planning and preparing nutritious meals customized to the individual's nutritional needs. Ensuring appropriate hydration and a balanced diet help not only physical health but also to the general well-being of stroke survivors. Mealtime becomes an occasion for sustenance and social engagement.

4. Communication Support:

Stroke survivors may face difficulty in communication, including difficulties with speech. Caregivers provide crucial help by utilizing approaches indicated by speech therapists, using communication aids, or just showing patience and understanding. Effective communication is crucial to addressing emotional and practical demands.

Medication Management at Home

1. Understanding Medication Regimens:

Many stroke survivors are administered drugs to treat chronic health concerns and avoid additional consequences. Caregivers have a vital role in knowing the recommended prescription regimes, including dosage, frequency, and any adverse effects. Clear contact with healthcare providers enables proper adherence to the specified plan.

2. Medication Organization:

Managing several drugs may be challenging. Caregivers help stroke survivors by collecting drugs in pill organizers, creating a timetable for administration, and assuring timely refills. This systematic method lowers the possibility of missed doses or prescription mistakes, enhancing the efficacy of the prescribed treatment.

3. Monitoring for Adverse Reactions:

Vigilance is key in drug management. Caregivers are vigilant to any symptoms of bad reactions or changes in the individual's health. Open contact with healthcare providers allows for fast revisions to the drug regimen if necessary. This coordinated approach guarantees that medicine contributes favorably to the rehabilitation path.

Monitoring for Signs of Complications

1. Regular Health Check ups:

Ongoing monitoring of health entails frequent check ups with healthcare specialists. Caregivers arrange these sessions, ensuring that any concerns or changes in health are adequately reported to the healthcare team. Routine checkups contribute to the early diagnosis of potential issues and the execution of prompt treatments.

2. Observing Physical and Cognitive Changes:

Caregivers are vigilant observers of physical and cognitive changes in stroke survivors. This includes monitoring for indicators of growing weakness, changes in movement, adjustments in speech or communication, and any indications of pain or discomfort. Early detection allows for quick action and modifications to the care plan.

3. Emotional Well-being:

The emotional well being of stroke survivors is crucial to their overall health. Caregivers offer emotional support, promote chances for social involvement, and encourage activities that bring joy and fulfillment. Monitoring for indicators of sadness or anxiety help caregivers to engage with healthcare experts to handle mental health concerns efficiently.

In the area of home care for stroke survivors, caregivers build a tapestry of care that incorporates physical safety, emotional well-being, and the preservation of freedom. The adaptations made to the living environment resound with a dedication to safety, while support with everyday tasks respects the individual's liberty. Medication management and watchful monitoring establish a complete framework for holistic assistance, addressing the multiple needs of stroke survivors on their road to recovery. The house, once adapted and nourished, becomes not merely a physical place but a sanctuary where healing and growth blossom with each passing day.

Support for Caregivers

As caregivers begin on the remarkable path of caring for stroke survivors, they become the unsung heroes, giving compassion, aid, and constant support. However, this duty may be emotionally and physically taxing, leading to caregiver stress. This section goes into the problems caregivers encounter, techniques for managing stress, and the necessity of obtaining help from healthcare experts and connecting with support groups and resources.

Understanding Caregiver Stress

1. The Weight of Caregiving:

Caregiving for a stroke survivor is a responsibility that comes with both joys and hardships. The physical responsibilities of aiding with everyday duties, coupled with the emotional effect of seeing a loved one's struggle, can produce a tremendous sense of obligation. Understanding the various stressors is the first step in reducing caregiver stress.

2. Emotional Impact:

Caregivers often experience a range of emotions, from empathy and affection to impatience and grief. Witnessing the changes in a loved one's skills and coping with the uncertainty of recovery may be emotionally exhausting. It's vital for caregivers to identify and affirm their sentiments as they manage the complexity of their position.

3. Balancing Act:

Caregivers typically find themselves balancing numerous duties — caretaker, advocate, and, in many circumstances, continuing with their career and personal commitments. This juggling act can lead to physical and emotional tiredness, underlining the need for self care and support.

Seeking Support from Healthcare Professionals

1. Open Communication:

Establishing open contact with healthcare experts is crucial for caregivers. This requires regular meetings with the stroke survivor's medical team to gather insights into the current health state, progress, and any revisions needed in the treatment plan. A collaborative approach ensures that caregivers feel knowledgeable and supported in their work.

2. Educational Resources:

Healthcare providers can provide caregivers with educational tools that increase their awareness of stroke recovery, possible complications, and techniques for successful care. Access to credible information helps caregivers to make educated decisions and actively engage in the healing path.

3. Training and Skill Development:

Caregivers may benefit from training programs that provide them with the required skills for delivering care. This may include instruction on mobility assistance, understanding prescription regimes, and managing assistive gadgets. Building caregiver competency helps to a sense of confidence in their caring position.

Connecting with Support Groups and Resources

1. Peer Support:

One of the most significant forms of support for caregivers is connecting with people who share similar experiences. Peer support groups provide a platform for caregivers to discuss their concerns, insights, and coping skills. The understanding and empathy within these organizations generate a feeling of community that combats the isolation that caregivers may experience.

2. Online Resources:

The internet realm offers a multitude of information for caregivers. Online forums, blogs, and social media groups dedicated to stroke care provide a venue for knowledge sharing and emotional support. Caregivers may obtain practical suggestions, success stories, and coping techniques offered by others who have walked a similar route.

3. Professional Counseling:

Recognizing the emotional toll of caregiving, some caregivers find relief in professional therapy. Mental health specialists can offer a safe environment for caregivers to express their emotions, handle feelings of guilt or fear, and create coping techniques. Counseling becomes a proactive element in sustaining the emotional well-being of caregivers.

4. Respite Care:

Caregivers may seek respite care choices, enabling them brief breaks from their caring obligations. This might entail requesting the support of friends, family members, or professional caregivers to step in temporarily, providing caregivers with the time to recharge and attend to their own needs.

Nurturing the Caregiver

In the complicated tapestry of stroke rehabilitation, caregivers are the threads that weave support, love, and understanding. Recognizing and managing caregiver stress is not only a humane gesture but also vital for preserving the caregiver's capacity to deliver appropriate care. Seeking help from healthcare experts ensures that caregivers are prepared with the information and skills essential for their task.

Connecting with support groups and resources increases the support network, delivering a collective knowledge formed from shared experiences. Caregivers, when nourished and encouraged, become pillars of strength, capable of weathering the trials of caregiving with fortitude and grace. As the caregiver receives the assistance they need, they, in turn, may provide more effective and compassionate care to the stroke survivor, establishing a symbiotic partnership that encourages overall well being for both.

Long-Term Outlook and Follow-Up Care

Nurturing Progress, Embracing Adaptation

As stroke survivors continue on the path to long-term recovery, the journey unfolds as a dynamic process, distinguished by progress, adaptation, and a dedication to sustained well being. This section delves into the essential elements of follow-up care and the long-term outlook. It highlights the need for regular follow-up appointments and checkups, the adaptive nature of care strategies to address changing needs, and the continuous monitoring and management of potential complications.

Monitoring and Managing Potential Complications

1. Vigilance in Health Monitoring:

Long-term care begins with a commitment to careful health monitoring. Stroke survivors, together with their healthcare team and caregivers, keep vigilant to any issues that may occur post-stroke. This involves regular examinations of cardiovascular health, brain function, and the effect of any concomitant health issues.

2. Addressing Cognitive Changes:

Cognitive health is a vital part of long-term care. Stroke survivors and their caregivers remain sensitive to any cognitive abnormalities, such as memory loss or trouble with thinking. Regular cognitive evaluations, generally completed during follow-up consultations, inform the application of interventions to enhance cognitive function and address new issues.

3. Management of Emotional Well being:

Emotional well being is essential to the long term outlook for stroke survivors. The emotional effect of a stroke may endure, and monitoring for indicators of anxiety, despair, or emotional distress is necessary. Collaborative efforts between healthcare experts, caregivers, and perhaps mental health specialists contribute to a complete approach to emotional well being.

Regular Check Ups and Follow Up Appointments

1. Frequency of Follow Up Appointments:

The frequency of follow up appointments may vary depending on the individual's health state and special needs. Initially, follow up sessions may be more frequent, allowing healthcare providers to closely monitor recovery progress and handle any acute issues. As time advances and stability is established, follow up sessions may become less frequent but remain an essential element of long term care.

2. Comprehensive Health Assessments:

Follow up consultations comprise detailed health examinations that continue beyond the immediate aftermath of the stroke. These exams involve cardiovascular health, neurological function, medication management, and emotional well being. They serve as a forum for open communication between the healthcare team, stroke survivors, and caregivers.

3. Adapting Care Plans:

The dynamic nature of healing needs an adaptable approach to care programs. Follow-up sessions give a chance to review the success of existing methods and make required improvements. This flexibility ensures that care plans fit with the developing requirements of the individual, fostering continuing growth and addressing any emergent obstacles.

Adjusting Care Strategies Based on Evolving Needs

1. Mobility and Rehabilitation:

Long term care entails a persistent focus on mobility and rehabilitation. As the individual develops in their recovery, rehabilitation treatments may change from intense interventions to maintenance and optimizing of mobility. This may require continual physical treatment, adaptive exercises, and the incorporation of assistive technologies based on developing needs.

2. Medication Management:

Medication management is a cornerstone of long term care. Follow up sessions give a platform for monitoring the efficacy of current drugs, modifying doses if needed, and addressing any new health issues. The objective is to optimize pharmaceutical regimens to prevent additional problems and enhance general well being.

3. Cognitive and Emotional Support:

Cognitive and emotional assistance continue to be crucial components of long term care. Care plans may involve continuing cognitive exercises, mental stimulation activities, and access to resources that enhance emotional well being. Regular assessments during follow up meetings encourage the customizing of support measures to correspond with the individual's growing cognitive and emotional demands.

4. Holistic Wellness:

The long term approach promotes holistic wellbeing covering physical, mental, and emotional well being. Care techniques may expand beyond typical medical procedures to include lifestyle adjustments, social involvement, and hobbies that offer joy and fulfillment. The integration of holistic wellness supports a complete approach to long term care that fosters the individual's entire quality of life.

Sustaining Hope, Encouraging Progress

Long term view and follow up care encompass the persistent commitment to optimism, progress, and continued well being. By monitoring and controlling possible complications, engaging in frequent check ups and follow up consultations, and modifying treatment plans based on growing requirements, stroke survivors, caregivers, and healthcare professionals cooperate in a journey distinguished by the resilience and continual improvement.

As the tapestry of recovery develops, the threads of care, support, and adaptability build a story of triumph over adversity. The long term prognosis becomes a canvas where each stroke survivor's tale is painted with the hues of progress, tenacity, and the steadfast confidence that, with continued care and devotion, the route of recovery is a path toward a satisfying and meaningful life.

Conclusion

As we pull the curtain on this complete guide to stroke care, we reflect on the rich tapestry woven with insights, techniques, and a caring knowledge of the issues encountered by stroke survivors and their caregivers. The road of stroke rehabilitation is distinguished by resilience, adaptation, and constant dedication to nurturing well-being. In this last piece, we highlight essential aspects, offer encouragement for caregivers, and share final views on stroke treatment and prevention.

Recap of Key Points

1. Understanding Strokes:

The course begins with an analysis of the intricacies of strokes, differentiating between ischemic and hemorrhagic strokes. It dug into the causes, risk factors, and the developing landscape of stroke research, including the potential relationship between COVID 19 and stroke risk.

2. Recognizing Stroke Symptoms:

Recognizing the indicators of a stroke evolved as a vital feature, with the FAST acronym acting as a mnemonic for fast response. Beyond the acronym, the guide emphasized other symptoms, highlighting the need for quick action and the impact of time on treatment success.

3. Medical Emergency and Initial Response:

Urgency in obtaining emergency medical aid, offering comfort, and explaining symptoms and medical history to healthcare specialists are important elements in the early reaction to a stroke.

4. Diagnosis and Treatment:

Diagnostic methods such as CT scans and MRIs, along with pharmacological therapies like clot busting medicines and anticoagulant medications, were studied. The part stressed the need for fast and correct diagnosis for optimal therapy.

5. Post Stroke Care:

Hospitalization, rehabilitation, medication management, and treating emotional and psychological elements comprised the foundations of post stroke treatment. The guide stressed the entire aspect of healing, embracing physical, mental, and emotional well being.

6. Lifestyle Modifications for Stroke Prevention:

Preventive approaches, including dietary guidelines, exercise, blood pressure control, smoking cessation, and alcohol moderation, were listed as critical techniques for minimizing the risk of stroke.

7. Home Care for Stroke Survivors:

Adapting the living environment for safety, aiding with daily tasks, administering medications at home, and monitoring for symptoms of problems were investigated in the context of home care for stroke survivors.

8. Support for Caregivers:

The specific problems encountered by caregivers were addressed, and solutions for managing caregiver stress, getting help from healthcare experts, and connecting with support groups were highlighted.

9. Long Term Outlook and Follow Up Care:

The dynamic aspect of long term rehabilitation, including the monitoring and treatment of possible problems, regular check ups, and the adaptive modification of care plans, was explored in the context of sustaining progress and well being.

Encouragement for Caregivers

To the caregivers who provide the basis of support for stroke survivors, we express our deepest appreciation and encouragement. Your work is both tough and crucial, and it's essential to acknowledge the strength inside you. As you manage the intricacies of caring, remember:

1. You Are Not Alone:

Reach out for help from healthcare experts, support groups, and resources. Understanding that you are not alone in your path will relieve the sense of loneliness that caring may sometimes bring.

2. Self Care Matters:

Prioritize self care to ensure you are equipped physically and emotionally.

Taking minutes for oneself is not selfish; it's a crucial component of preserving your capacity to offer excellent care.

3. Adaptability is a Strength:

The road of stroke recovery is dynamic, and your capacity to adjust to shifting demands is a tribute to your strength. Embrace the process of adaptation, understanding that flexibility is an important ability in caregiving.

4. Celebrate Small Victories:

Each milestone, no matter how minor, is an accomplishment worth celebrating. Whether it's a physical success, a cognitive milestone, or a moment of emotional connection, these wins add to the overall advancement.

5. Communication is Key:

Maintain open contact with healthcare experts and establish a collaborative partnership. Your insights into the daily realities of stroke survivors are crucial for improving and enhancing treatment programs.

Final Thoughts on Stroke Care and Prevention

In our last discussion of stroke treatment and prevention, we appreciate the leaps achieved in medical breakthroughs, the perseverance of individuals on the path of recovery, and the devotion of caregivers. Our ideas converge on the significance of a comprehensive strategy that incorporates medical treatments, lifestyle adjustments, and a solid support network.

Preventing strokes takes a community effort, from individuals making aware choices to healthcare professionals giving information and support. The road of stroke recovery, while defined by hardships, is also a monument to the tenacious spirit of the human will.

As we complete this guide, let us carry on the knowledge, compassion, and commitment to promoting a future where strokes are prevented, and those afflicted receive thorough and compassionate treatment. May the echoes of support resound, and the waves of improvement continue to touch the lives of stroke survivors and their caregivers.

In the mosaic of stroke treatment, each contribution, each attempt, constitutes a part of a bigger narrative—a narrative of hope, healing, and the triumph of the human spirit.